Our Family Doctor

A Companion to "Our Household Medicine Case";
The ABC of Medicine, Especially Adapted to Daily
Use in the Home

(19th Century Medical History)

By Orville W. Owen

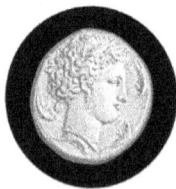

PANTIANOS
CLASSICS

Published by Pantianos Classics

ISBN-13: 978-1-78987-097-8

First published in 1887

Contents

Disclaimer

The contents of this book represent medical diagnoses, procedures and treatments dating to the late nineteenth century. The publisher does not condone, advise or assume any responsibility for this book's use in any medical context.

The contents herein are presented purely and solely for informational and historical purposes.

Publishers' Preface (1887)

THE preparation of the present little volume was undertaken by the publishers in response to what appeared to them a real demand for such a work — alike brief, comprehensive, intelligible, cheap, and — so far as possible, within what seemed to them the proper limits of a work, intended for every-day household use — complete. The book, as its title page indicates, is signed for family use, and is such a work as is frequently to be resorted to in cases of great exigency when *dispatch* is a main consideration, and there is little time and inclination for the hazardous delays requisite for reading through long pages of learned medical discussion — all right in its proper place, perhaps, but that place *not* in a medical adviser and guide-book *for the laity only.* The work is also a companion (and a key) to "Our Household Medicine Case," a package of standard medicines of the greatest purity, prepared expressly for us by one of the best and most favorably known wholesale drug houses of the West.

Works bearing the pretentious titles of "Family Physician," "Domestic Doctor," "Household Medical Adviser," "Hand Book of Medicine," etc., etc., were plentiful enough before, and many, if not most, of these possessed merits of their own; but they were and are, one and all, voluminous, huge tomes, containing the germ of truth within them often, but with such envelopment of husk that it lay (and lies) like the traditional "needle in the hay stack," so difficult to discover that frequently, ere the particular remedy sought was found, the patient for whose benefit the search had been instituted, had died — or recovered — and (in either case, let us hope) gone on his way rejoicing!

A further difficulty was always found: When the symptoms of the patient's complaint had been gathered, as with a skimmer, from a very dilute and watery stream of discourse, and the proper remedy had been made out, the materials wherewith to compound the potion were not at hand, but were at the distant drug store! What wonder at the result when, in nine cases out of ten, with all the danger and damage — to be charged to the profit and loss account — in the end the guardians of the poor sufferer, — in whose case ominous changes begin to develop during the terrible delay, — throw aside the lumbering medical volume with a secret anathema upon the heads of its unfortunate author and publisher, and hurry at last to the doctor whose task has perhaps by this time grown far too huge for him! Then the good doctor arrives: notes the patient's symptoms, and decides on the remedies. But doctors do not carry a drug store with them, and now a second trip — and an expensive one, too, — becomes requisite, before which has been completed who can compute what valuable moments shall be lost, what irreparable and long-to-be-lamented injury may often result!

The publishers would respectfully request the reader's attention to the following considerations, viz:

With the present combination of the brief but comprehensive work, couched in the plainest and simplest language (so that a child may read and reading may understand), with this medicine case filled with all the ordinarily used and standard remedies, we furnish you *at about one-half the usual price demanded for the book alone* (designed to fill but poorly the place our book fills so well) *both a medical guide-book and the remedies prescribed.*

Our book is written by one of the most successful and best known of the younger physicians of our State, a man thoroughly educated in his profession, acquainted with all the remedies and appliances known thereto, and withal thoroughly conscientious and scrupulously exact in every statement of his pen. Hence we claim our work to be simpler, more complete (although comparatively so brief), cheaper and *safer* than any other extant.

Our medicines are purer (and hence safer), cheaper, and better than can be ordinarily obtained elsewhere, being prepared expressly for us in large quantities by a wholesale house of unexcelled reputation, whose sworn statement accompanies every case.

We claim without fear of successful contradiction that with this arrangement we make it wholly practicable for a large majority of the cases of incipient disease that arise to be promptly handled and *cured by strictly home management,* whereby great pain and anxiety will be avoided, vast pecuniary expense spared, yea, and which will often result in the saving of life!

The public everywhere who have tested our system are cheerfully giving in their testimony to its inestimable value, and many intelligent persons have gone so far as to declare that the beneficent thought in which it originated **was a real inspiration!**

Author's Introduction

The author makes no apology for placing this little book and accompanying medicine case before the public. He believes it is a necessity in every household in the land. It has been written not for the profit arising from its sale, but for the purpose of teaching the people how to treat and doctor the common diseases of every day life: to accomplish this no technical terms or medical words have been used, but only plain, old-fashioned English. All the remedies are standard ones and are put up under the author's own personal supervision, and are as tasteless as it is possible to make them. Where whisky, brandy or other liquors are prescribed they are the only stimulants which could be used, and they would have most certainly been left out if any other remedy or remedies could have been substituted.

In conclusion, if this little volume with its companion medicine case, shall cure but one who is sick, or alleviate one painful symptom, or help some mother to save her loved child, then its work will have been accomplished and its end obtained, and if it does as much good to those who buy it as it has given pleasure to the author in its writing, then I say unto it, God speed, and send it on its way rejoicing.

Orville W. Owen, M. D.,
22 Lafayette Avenue.

July 15, 1886.

Special Notice

OUR facilities enable us to furnish all varieties of *Standard Drugs and Medicines,* in solid form (by mail, *postpaid,* to any part of the United States), on request, *at unusually low rates.* Orders by mail solicited. Particularly are we desirous of replenishing, when low, the stock of family remedies we furnish the purchasers of "Our Household Medicine Case" and this little book, for we are solicitous that this store shall be kept up from *pure and reliable medicines,* as we guarantee they shall be if obtained of us.

Detroit Medicine Co.,
22 Lafayette Ave., Detroit, Mich.

This Book is Respectfully Dedicated
to the
Faithful Wives and Mothers of This Country,
With a Heartfelt Wish for their
Welfare,

by

The Author

Our Family Doctor

The Normal or Healthy Condition

Temperature, 98 ½ by fever thermometer; pulse, adult, 72 per minute; new born, 124 to 160 per minute; 1st month to close of 3d month, 112 to 148 per minute; close of 3d month to close of 6th month, 112 to 146 per minute: from 6th month to close of 1st year, 112 to 144 per minute; from close of 1st to 3d year, 90 to 112.

Respiration or Breathing

1st week, 52; 1st month, 59; 2d and 3d months, 51; 3d to 6th months, 50; 6th month to 1 year, 41. All these are per minute. The adult breathes about 18 times per minute.

Bronchitis

Symptoms: — Sneezing, running at the nose, headache, flushed face, fever, fast pulse, (120 per minute or more) slight cough which increases, fretfulness, loss of appetite, fast breathing, spittle frothy and sometimes bloody. Duration of disease, 3 to 15 days. *Dangerous!*

Treatment: — Apply mustard poultice to the lungs until flesh is very red, then apply hot flax seed poultices every hour. Give Carbonate of Ammonia. For child 3 months old, one tablet in teaspoonful of water every 3 hours; child 6 to 12 months old, one tablet in "water every one and one-half hours; adult, one tablet in water every half hour, For the fever in children one year old, give one-half tablet of Aconite in water every 15 minutes until patient sweats, then stop. For adults, give 1 tablet of Aconite every 15 minutes until sweating occurs, then stop. If there is much sinking, give whisky in doses of ½ to 4 teaspoonfuls every hour. For weak heart action, give ½ tablet of Digitalis in water every 2 hours for child one year old; for adults, 1 tablet every hour; if the pulse is strong or irregular, stop the Digitalis.

Pneumonia — Lung Fever

There are two kinds, Catarrhal Pneumonia and Croupous Pneumonia.

Catarrhal Pneumonia

Symptoms: — Usually occurs with other diseases or in the course of other troubles such as Measles or Whooping Cough. High fever with remissions, skin may perspire freely, pulse frequent but may become irregular, breathing frequent and labored, cough hacking and painful, patient tries to hold it back, spittle hardly ever "rusty" in color, (See Croupous Pneumonia) patient may become stupid, lips blue, nostrils dilated, great loss of strength and fat, restlessness, recovery slow, very dangerous disease.

Treatment: — Give 1 tablet of Ipecac and 1 tablet of Muriate of Ammonia every hour to adult, ½ tablet of Ipecac and ½ tablet of Muriate of Ammonia to child 5 to 10 years old. for child 6 months to five years old dissolve 1 tablet of Ipecac and 1 tablet of Muriate of Ammonia in 4 teaspoonfuls of water and give 1 teaspoonful every hour or two, apply flaxseed poultices over the whole lungs in both children and adults. Where there is much sinking give Carbonate of Ammonia in wine or whisky without stint; when the lungs are badly loaded up as shown by the heavy breathing, crowd the Ipecac until vomiting takes place.

Croupous Pneumonia

Symptoms: — Usually commences very suddenly, fever high, restlessness, vomiting, headache, may have delirium, pain in the side which usually comes on with the chill, chill is marked, very rapid breathing and has the "expiratory moan," that is as the air leaves the lungs the patient moans; cough commences early, is short and hacking and often comes on in spasms, spittle becomes "rusty," that is red like iron rust and is so sticky that it is hard to get it out of the mouth and it will stick to the 1 even when the vessel is reversed, after a time the spittle becomes yellow, then white; urine is scanty and high colored, skin hot and dry, having a burning feel to the hand; fever high on second or third day with a daily variation, lowest in the morning, tongue dry and furred, lips crack, may have vomiting and inability to swallow, thirst marked, may have matter form in the lungs, water blisters may appear on the face, lasts from 3 to 11 days; moderately dangerous.

Treatment: — The main treatment is to keep up the patient's strength. Do this by giving soups, wine or brandy and give 1 Carbonate of Ammonia tablet in teaspoonful of water every hour to adult, or ½ or ¼ tablet of Carbonate of Ammonia to children. Children arc not very subject to Croupous Pneumonia.

Pleurisy

Symptoms: — Chills at beginning, pain below nipple or under the arm, which is very sharp and stitch-like; pain increased by breathing or coughing; breathing fast, 30 to 35 per minute; irregular and shallow — that is, the lungs are not filled full of air, on account of the pain — cough generally present, patient tries not to cough on account of pain, at first patient will lie on sore side, fever not very high, pulse 90 to 120 per minute, full, strong and bounding, headache. Matter may form in lung; when this happens the patient wastes away, hair falls out, ends of fingers become "clubbed," skin becomes hot, dry and harsh; pulse weak. Disease is moderately dangerous.

Treatment: — Strap the painful side; get some long, adhesive plaster strips; commence on the back, at the spine, and stick one end to the flesh, then bring the strip around to the front, where it should end in middle of chest, and a little lower down than where it was started. The first strip should be put on about 2 ½ inches below the nipple, and the others put above this, until the chest is about half covered; the strips should be about 1 inch wide. A tightly bound cloth bandage will do in place of strips, but is not as good, as it has to be wound around the whole body. Give 1 tablet of Opium every hour to adult, to relieve pain, or, dissolve 1 Morphine tablet in 4 teaspoonfuls of water, and give ½ teaspoonful every hour to child 5 to 10 years old, to relieve pain. Dissolve 1 tablet of Aconite in 4 teaspoonfuls of water, and give 2 teaspoonfuls every half hour to adults till sweating occurs, then stop. Give 1 teaspoonful of the Aconite and water every half hour, to child 5 to 10 years old, till sweating occurs, then stop. When you are sure you have Pleurisy, and after 24 hours of the above treatment without any benefit, send for your doctor.

Colds

Symptoms: — Sneezing, slight cough, running at the nose, watery eyes, furred tongue, diarrhoea, or constipation, slight headache, pain in the limbs and back, comes on gradually. Do not let it run, as it may become a serious trouble.

Treatment: — Dissolve 1 tablet of Morphine in 8 teaspoonfuls of water; add to this 1 tablet of Carbonate of Ammonia, and 1 tablet of Ipecac. For child 3 to 5 years old, ½ teaspoonful every 2 hours; for child 5 to 10 years old, 1 teaspoonful every 2 hours. To adult, 2 teaspoonfuls every 15 minutes to half hour. Grease the nose and between the eyes with Vaseline, and open the bowels with a compound Cathartic pill, for the grown people, and 1 tablet of Calomel every hour, for the children. You can leave out the Morphine, if you wish.

Small Pox — Variola

Symptoms: — From 10 to 13 days after exposure to small pox the patient begins to have the chill, backache, headache and fever, which ushers in this horrible dis: the fever is high, 104 to 105 degrees from the start and with it the pulse jumps up to 120 to 140 per minute. Vomiting and sick stomach, with sore throat are now prominent symptoms; light-headedness by the 2nd day is a common feature. After three days of the fever the '"rash" or better, eruption comes on, this first appears as slightly elevated red points, about as large as a pin-head or millet seed, and are movable and hard; they make their appearance first on the forehead, nose and lips; they slowly increase in size and burn and itch; in about 12 hours after they have appeared on the face, the body, arms and legs, then the hands and feet are covered; the points will be found on the *inside of the hands and bottom of feet, the only eruption doing this.* On the second day after the eruption appears, the spots or points turn a darker red and become elevated above the skin; on the third day they are pointed slightly and have a little water blister on top; they are now about the size of a small pea; as they now enlarge a depression or cup forms on their top which looks like the naval (umbilicated.) When the eruption is out, all the other symptoms subside; fever falls and pulse is slower; about the 6th day of the eruption matter commences to form in the water blisters, and by the 8th day the pock is complete. Around the pock or pustule, the skin becomes red, swollen and angry looking, the face swells to a large size and the itching is fearful; during this stage the odor of the room is sickening. From the evening of the 8th or 9th day of the eruption the pock commences to grow smaller and dries up and by the 14th day they commence to fall off, leaving the pits which are red in color, and if the pock has been ruptured by scratching the pit is deep and will never disappear except in very young children. On the 8th day you will have the secondary fever, which generally commences with a chill; when the crusts fall off this fever disappears.

This is a very dangerous disease and should always be treated by a skillful doctor. It is catching, and no one but the nurse should be allowed in the room.

Treatment: — For severe headache put cold packs on head; give iced milk as food and when the sinking stage is reached, which is sure to come, dissolve 2 tablets of Carbonate of Ammonia in 1 tablespoonful of brandy and give it every hour, or oftener if needed, open each x on the face and hands as soon as the water blister forms and keep cloths dipped in cold water over the this stops the itching and saves the pitting. Always have your children vaccinated every 5 years as it is the only sure way of preventing small pox. Never give a cathartic.

Chicken-Pox

Symptoms: — Slight fever, headache, chill, languor, sometimes back and limb ache. Pulse 100 to 112 per minute. In 24 hours, eruption, or pocks appear, first on body, then on face and limbs. The pocks are small, red, and have water in them, the water appears in the whole of the spots at th*e same time*; there is no depression or hardness to the pock, and no regular size. (See Small Pox.) *No danger.*

Treatment: — Bromide of Potash, 1 tablet in 10 teaspoonfuls of water, 1 teaspoonful every 2 to 3 hours.

Scarlet Fever — Scarlatina

Symptoms: — A contagious or catching disease, comes on within 6 to 8 days after exposure, within 24 to 48 hours after the child is taken sick rash appears which lasts from 5 to 9 days, then the "peeling" or throwing off the dead skin commences which lasts a longer or shorter period, generally about 8 days. The child may be and generally is, taken sick suddenly, commences to vomit, has flushed face, sore throat, tongue red and looks like a strawberry, chilliness, pulse fast, fever, thirst, neck stiff, joints tender, then in 24 or 48 hours as a rule you will find a fine red rash coming out, which itches badly; it first appears on the neck and upper part of the chest, this fine rash runs together and extends over the whole body, face and limbs. On the fourth day after the rash appears if you draw your thumb nail along the rash a white line appears which lasts for some time. After the second day of the rash the whole surface of the child will be covered. Perhaps a flea bite looks the nearest like a scarlet fever rash. The color varies according to the severity of the disease, the darker red it is the more severe will be the sickness. The dangers are many in scarlet fever and consist of diphtheria with the scarlet fever, matter forming at angle of the jaw, brain trouble from the disease going to the brain, kidney trouble, which brings on swelling of the hands and feet, trouble with the eyes and lungs.

Treatment: — Keep the patient warm in bed from the start to the very end, about 3 weeks, for a cold while the child is "peeling," will nearly always kill it. Keep the rash greased, as this gives comfort, and when peeling commences, keeps the skin from blowing about. Give cool drinks, not too cold, and dissolve 3 tablets of Tincture of Iron in 8 teaspoonfuls of water, add 6 tablets of Sulphur, 4 tablets of Chlorate of Potash, and 8 Quinine pills; dissolve them all together, and give Y 2 teaspoonful of this mixture every three hours to child 1 to 3 years old; 1 teaspoonful every 3 hours to child 3 to 6 years old, and 1 ½ teaspoonfuls every 3 hours to child 6 to 12 years old. If the child has spasms, put it in a hot mustard bath, and apply ice to back of head. Never give a Cathartic in scarlet fever, measles, German measles, small pox or chicken pox. Give light foods, without spices in them, and keep the other children, and neighbors, out of the room and house. The dangers or complications of scarlet fever, should only be treated by a skillful physician, and for that reason I do not give their treatment.

Measles

Symptoms: — More frequent or more common than any of the other contagious or catching diseases, 8 or 10 days after exposure, the child begins to have snuffles, running at the eyes and nose, feels tired, chilly and fretful, may have some fever, light hurts the eyes, pain in forehead, slight sore throat, dry cough, the whites of the eyes become very red and inflamed; this is characteristic of Measles; fever rises, and in from 2 to 5 days the rash appears, first upon the face, then neck, then upon the chest, body and limbs. It takes about 4 days for it to go over the whole body and extremities. The rash comes on in fine, red dots or points, which run together, and form half moon shape patches, the skin between them being natural in color, differing from scarlet fever in this respect; with the rash the skin becomes swollen, and burns and itches, the eruption or rash reaches its height about the end of the third day from its appearance, and then commences to turn yellow and fade, and generally entirely gone by the end of the 6th day. Sneezing, coughing, and fever are very marked during the rash. Pulse 100 to 120 per minute, fever 106 to 107 degrees; as soon as the rash begins to disappear, the fever falls, and all the symptoms abate in violence. The skin of the child now peels off, but not nearly as much as in scarlet fever. This is not a dangerous disease, unless complications set in, such as Bronchitis, Pneumonia, Ear and Eye inflammations, (see these diseases), Kidney, Brain or intestinal troubles. Diphtheria is not a very common complication with Measles.

Treatment: — Keep the patient warm, give warm drinks till the rash appears; Dissolve 1 tablet of Chlorate of Potash in 6 teaspoonfuls of water, give 1 teaspoonful every hour or two till throat symptoms subside. Put 1 tablet of Sulphate of Zinc in a half pint of warm water and wash the eyes out every 4 to 6 hours, keep the room dark, and grease the patient to keep down the itching. If fever is very high give 1 Quinine pill every 4 hours to child 5 to 10 years old, ½ Quinine pill every 4 hours to child 1 to 5 years old; keep the room at 79° temperature, give light food. If the child has the ear-ache pour hot water in the ear with a tablespoon every 15 minutes and use at least 6 of the tablespoonfuls of water at a time, use the water as hot as it can be borne by the child.

German Measles – Rötheln

Symptoms: — The child feels sick from 12 to 24 hours, when a light red rash appears, which may first appear on the back, chest, cheeks or neck; it is in round patches and may look like measles or scarlet fever. I have seen cases where the cheeks, neck and chest looked exactly like measles, and on the arms and legs of the same child the rash had all the appearance of scarlet fever. A mild in-flammation is noticed of the eyes and throat, fever is usually mild and pulse about 100 per minute, only a few of the children have cough, tongue is usually covered with a light fur, slight vomiting may occur, no ger at present, but I believe as the disease becomes more common that it will in time be a very dangerous

Treatment: — Keep the child warm, give warm drinks; dissolve 1 tablet of Chlorate of Potash in 10 teaspoonsful of water, and give 1 teaspoonful every 3 or 4 hours till throat is well. Keep patient in a dark room and give plain food without meats.

Erysipelas. — The Rose, St. Anthony's Fire.

Symptoms: — There are two kinds, one coming from wounds, bites and scratches, the other a blood disease; both kinds are catch-ing. May commence on any part of the body, legs, arms, face or neck. Restlessness from pain, which is burning, and comes on as soon as the skin becomes red. High fever, difficult breathing com-mon in children, chilliness, sore throat, bowels loose, as a rule, though they may be bound up; nose-bleed common, skin feels hot, tight and dry, tender to the touch, becomes red, swollen, firm, tense and shining; redness starts from one spot and slowly spreads, usually in one direction; as the disease goes on, the color becomes darker, swelling becomes greater, and will pit or depress under pressure; pulse full, strong, and 100 to 120 per minute, worse in evening. The redness may jump from one place to another on the surface of the body, or may go to the brain, may form matter. Dangerous disease, and nearly always kills children.

Treatment: — Cool drinks, good food, cranberry poultices, put on hot. Dissolve 1 tablet of Tincture of Iron in a teaspoonful of water, and give it every 1 or 2 hours to a grown person; for children, 1 tablet of the Iron in 5 teaspoonfuls of sweetened water, and give ½ teaspoonful every 2 to 3 hours to child 1 to 5 years old; 1 teaspoonful to child 5 to 10 years old. Give 1 Quinine pill every 2 hours to grown person; 1 Quinine pill every 4 hours to child 5 to 10; ½ Quinine pill every 4 hours to child 1 year old. If there is much pain, give 1 Opium tablet to grown person every half hour, or dissolve 1 Morphine tablet in 10 teaspoonfuls of water and give 1 teaspoonful every half hour to child 5 to 10 years old; ¼ teaspoonful every hour to child 1 to 5 years old, till quiet, then stop.

Diphtheria

Symptoms: — At first, chilliness, slight headache, pain in back and legs, poor appetite, slight tenderness in throat, fever marked, tongue is moist, slight fur, patient may vomit, small lumps appear at angle of the jaw, inside of throat red, except where patch will appear, where the color is *bluish*; in 24 or more hours, a white membrane will commence to form on this blue spot, this membrane will soon turn slightly yellow and the breath will become offensive; may now have paralysis of throat, cannot swallow, pulse fast, spittle runs from mouth, face slightly flushed, tongue nasty, pain in swallowing, patch grows larger, and child begins to sink, urine becomes scanty, sweating profuse. Dangerous disease; one out of three generally die. Remember this disease is catching.

Treatment: — Put 3 tablets of the Tincture of Iron in 8 teaspoonfuls of water, add to this 8 tablets of Sulphur, 8 tablets of Chlorate of Potash, and 8 Quinine pills, dissolve them all together, and to child 1 year old give ½ teaspoonful of this mixture every 3 hours; to child 2 to 4 yrs old, 1 teaspoonful every 2 hours; to child 5 to 10 years old, 2 teaspoonfuls every 2 hours. After the 2nd day give wine or whisky, as much as is needed to keep the child from sinking. With the above medicines you can make the best right for your child's life. Do not be afraid to crowd the medicine, as your child is in a very dangerous condition, and you should keep the other children, and neighbors, out of the room, and send for your doctor.

Quinsy— Tonsillitis.

Symptoms: — Sore throat; on looking at the inside of throat one or both tonsils will be found swollen, red and full, tongue coated with fur, sides of and back of throat red and inflamed, tenderness behind the jaw, hurts to swallow, breathing may be difficult, voice altered and husky, snore loud when asleep, fever high, bowels bound up, great dryness of mouth with thirst, headache, restlessness, may have delirium at night, may have matter form in one or both tonsils, and if they are not lanced will break themselves and constitute the only danger, which is from suffocation; not a very dangerous disease.

Treatment: — Open up the bowels with salts, oil or Cathartic pills; give 1 Quinine pill every hour to adult till 12 have been taken, ½ Quinine pill every 3 hours to child 5 to 14 years old; dissolve 6 tablets Tincture of Iron in ½ glass of water, add 3 tablets of Belladonna and let an adult or children old enough, gargle the throat every hour spitting out the gargle when done. Heat water in a teakettle and allow the patient to breathe the hot steam as warm as can be borne; for young children who cannot gargle, put 2 tablets of

Tincture of Iron in 10 teaspoonfuls of water, add 5 Sulphur tablets and give ½ to 1 teaspoonful every hour according to the age of child, let the patient suck ice and bind salt pork around the neck.

Common Sore Throat

Symptoms: — Comes on suddenly, hurts to swallow, whole throat red and inflamed, bowels constipated, slight headache, tongue dirty, voice husky, may be deaf, pulse 100 to 120 per minute, some fever. No danger.

Treatment: — Open the bowels with oil, salts or compound cathartic pills, and give 1 tablet of Chlorate of Potash every hour until the throat is better.

Croup

There are two kinds, called "True Croup" and "False Croup."

False Croup

Symptoms: — Cough for two or three days, running at the nose, slight cold at first; or these symptoms may be absent. Between 10 and 12 o'clock at night may occur a sudden, loud, barking cough, whistling breathing, breathing hard, face flushed, great restlessness, skin hot and dry, pulse fast, lasts from 1 to three hours; patient generally gets well, — subject to return of disease.

Treatment: — Hot bath. Give 1 tablet of Ipecac in water every 20 minutes, till child vomits, keep warm; apply heat to neck. Next day give 1 Quinine pill every 4 hours, to child 2 years old.

True Croup

Symptoms: — Cold in head; hoarse, dry cough; voice hoarse, spittle frothy, membrane comes off when child vomits, breathing rapid, and the chest is quiet, the breathing being done by the bowel muscles; nostrils dilated, spasms of throat, and child throws itself from side to side; eyes wild, face anxious, fingers and lips blue, between spasms of throat, child is quiet; pulse, 110 to 190. If symptoms lull, do not think child is better, for usually they will recommence. Disease lasts from 2 to 14 days, and 19 out of 20 *die*.

Treatment: — Give 1 tablet of Ipecac in water every 20 minutes till vomiting occurs, then 1 tablet of Calomel every hour, until your doctor can get there, and send for him quick.

Hooping, or Whooping Cough

Symptoms: — A catching or contagious disease, generally caught in childhood, between the ages of 1 and 2 years; has 3 stages: 1st stage, sneezing, cough and mild bronchitis, eyes slightly red, no spittle; this stage may last from 3 days to 6 weeks. The 2nd stage then sets in, child feels a tickling in throat, which brings on a spasm of coughing, with tight feeling across the chest; child will put its head on its mother's knees or takes hold of some fixed thing to help it during the 'coughing; pulse and breathing during the spasm are slightly faster; the sound during the spasm of coughing is called the "hoop" or "whoop." The face becomes flushed during this period; as soon a3 the coughing is over, the child's face, pulse and breathing become natural again; the child will spit out a little frothy mucus; anger, fright or exertion will bring on the cough. This stage lasts until about the 35th day of the disease, when the 3rd stage sets in. Spittle turns yellow and is thicker, cough becomes less and is neither so frequent or so hard; child begins to breathe better during spasm and is getting well; this stage lasts for a longer or shorter period; sometimes 2 years after, if the child gets angered or frightened a spasm of coughing takes place. There is not much danger in this disease, unless complications set in, such as convulsions, bursting blood vessel, bronchitis or pneumonia; these, however, are rare.

Treatment: — During 1st stage, give 1 tablet of Muriate of Ammonia every 2 to 5 hours, keep child warm, and treat convulsions as directed (see Convulsions.) During 2nd stage or spasmodic cough, dissolve 2 tablets of Bromide of Potash in 10 teaspoonfuls of water, add 1 tablet of Opium and give 1 teaspoonful every 2 hours, or oftener if spasm is hard, to child 1 to 5 years old; in addition to this, dissolve one tablet of Belladonna in a teaspoonful of water and give it morning and evening until the spasms of coughing are controlled. During the 3rd stage no medicines are needed.

Mumps

Symptoms: — A catching or contagious disease; swelling and tenderness at one or both angles of jaw; this gradually increases until it fills all the space back to the ear and forward on the cheek; may have vomiting, pain in swallowing, especially anything sour; fever, which lasts about 48 hours; talking is painful, lasts from 8 to 10 days. Danger is the flying of disease to the ovaries of females and testicles of males.

Treatment: — Keep warm, stay in the house, and cover the swelling with cotton batting; give warm drinks. No medicine is needed. Do not take cold.

Cerebro-Spinal Fever — Or Spotted Fever.

Symptoms: — Commences between 12 A.M. and 6 A.M.; sudden attack, slight chill, or, in children, perhaps a spasm; unconsciousness, or delirium; violent pain in back of head and neck, vomiting usual, fever high at start, dizziness, restlessness, skin painful when touched, head drawn backward after one to two days, tongue coated white or brown, appetite gone, usually constipation, pulse 100 to 160 per minute, breathing quiet, skin white or pallid, goose flesh, dusky red or bluish spots, sometimes water blisters; cross eyes, deafness and loss of smell common — *generally a fatal disease!*

Treatment: — Give one tablet of Bromide of Potash in water every hour, ice-packs to head. For pain, 1 tablet of Morphine in 5 teaspoonfuls of water, 1 teaspoonful every half hour to child 1 year to 5 years old, 2 teaspoonfuls to child 5 to 10 years old, and 1 tablet to adult, till quiet, then stop the morphine.

Convulsions or Spasms

Symptoms: — Twitching and jerking of the limbs, frothing at mouth, grinding teeth, drawing up of legs and arms, clenched hands, with thumbs on the palms, eyes rolling or fixed, short breathing, head drawn back. Generally commencement of some other disease.

Treatment: — Put child into a hot mustard bath. Apply cold to top and back of head. Give one tablet of Bromide of Potash in one teaspoonful of sweetened water every half hour till quiet.

Congestion of Brain

Symptoms: — Common in childhood, though it may come on at any time of life; may come on of itself or during other diseases; stupor, insensibility, heat of head, throbbing of blood vessels, restlessness, when wakened twitching of limbs, convulsions, light hurts the eyes, not much fever or none at all, eyes bloodshot; dangerous disease.

Treatment: — Give one Calomel tablet every hour dry on the tongue till 12 have been taken, then give Salts till the bowels have moved thoroughly. If there is stupor at first give 1 tablet of Ipecac every 15 minutes till vomiting occurs then follow with the Calomel and Salts. Shave the head and apply ice all over the head, and send for your doctor.

Neuralgia

Symptoms: — May be located in any part of the body, sharp, shooting, tearing or dull pain, not much fever except from pain. People who are subject to neuralgia rarely ever become fully cured, and its treatment is very unsatisfactory both to patient and physician.

Treatment: — Give 1 tablet of Morphine every hour to grown person till pain is relieved, then stop. Apply hot poultices or cloths wrung out of hot water to the affected spot; pressure over the seat of pain will sometimes give relief; during the intervals of pain open the bowels with a Cathartic pill and give 1 Quinine pill every hour to adult, if the pain is in the jaw have the teeth examined by a good dentist. Electricity and rubbing or massage will sometimes give relief.

Rheumatism

Symptoms: — Acute Rheumatism occurs suddenly; it fever at first, becoming more marked, pain and redness of the joints which become swollen, may form matter, pulse 120 to 140 per minute, great sweating, appetite poor, tongue coated, bowels bound up, urine red, small amount and smells bad. If the Rheumatism leaves the joints and goes to the heart it is a very dangerous disease. It lasts about 14 days; you should have a doctor see the patient from time to time.

Treatment: — Cover the joint or joints afflicted, with cotton batting, over which bind flannel cloth and 1 Quinine pill every hour to adult, 1 Quinine pill every 3 hours to child 5 to 10 years old, and ½ Quinine pill every 3 hours to child 1 to 5 years old, when pain is excessive give adult 1 Morphine tablet every hour till quiet, then stop; to child dissolve 3 tablets of Bromide of Potash and 5 Muriate of Ammonia tablets in 5 teaspoonfuls of sweetened water and give 1 teaspoonful every 2 hours to children 1 to 10 years old. If pain goes to heart send for your doctor at once.

Cholera Infantum

Symptoms: — Generally abrupt, in beginning may have had diarrhoea, passages thin, frequent, watery like urine, odor musty; vomiting frequent, appetite gone, great thirst, tongue clean or light white fur, pulse fast, fever high, no pain, urine scanty, marked loss of strength and fat, eyes sunken, lips blue, restlessness, skin may feel cool, and lies in folds, child will not move to keep flies from eyes or face, lasts from 1 to 3 days. *Very dangerous!*

Treatment: — Dissolve 1 Morphine tablet in 4 teaspoonfuls of water, add 4 Bismuth tablets to this. Give a teaspoonful every hour to child 1 year old, every ½ hour to child 1 to 3 years old. If there is rolling of the head, or stupor, leave out the Morphine and give the Bismuth alone. When the stools are checked use the Bismuth alone. *Remember, Morphine is dangerous!* For the thirst, give pounded ice, and put cold packs at back of head. For the extreme weakness give 10 to 15 drops of brandy in a very little water every hour.

Cholera Morbus

Symptoms: — Comes on in 1 to 2 days with diarrhoea, usually griping pain in bowels, exhaustion, trembling, depression, have the blues, dizzy headed, pain in stomach, then the passages commence to increase in number, vomiting, great thirst, passages watery, looks like water in which rice has been boiled, sometimes a little blood in them; may have complete absence of pain, the vomit becomes yellow and green; cramps of the limbs, fingers and toes, now set in, and are fearful; now comes the stage of collapse, face pinched, lead colored or blue, eye-balls sunk back, eyes half open, nose looks pinched, skin of feet and hands wrinkled, pulse feeble, brain becomes stupid, no spittle, no urine. If this disease is very hard, it is so near real cholera that only the regular doctor can tell the difference. It is a very dangerous disease.

Treatment: — As soon as Diarrhoea appears, give 1 tablet of Calomel and 1 tablet of Morphine every half hour. The time to avert this disease is at the start. If, however, it has gone too long, give 1 tablet of Morphine, 1 tablet of Opium, and 1 tablet of Bromide of Potash every half hour till passages are cheeked. If. however, sinking and depression, with cold sweat, has commenced, do not give either the Morphine or the Opium, but give 1 tablet of Bromide of Potash, with 5 tablets of Carbonate of Bismuth every 20 minutes. Apply hot poultices to the bowels, and give the sick person ice to suck. Remember, do not let the disease get a start, and give the Opium and Morphine at once, as above, when there is only *slight* depression or collapse. Send for your doctor.

Dysentery — Bloody Flux

Symptoms: — Chill, thirst, fever, diarrhoea, colic, appetite gone, griping pains, twisting pain in bowels, heat bowels, tenderness on left side in groin, gas in bowels, bearing down pain in rectum, pain relieved after age, passages scanty, bloody, odor bad like carrion, may have hard lumps in them which look like raw meat, desire to pass water often, furred tongue, water high colored and smells bad. Lasts variable time. Dangerous disease, may become chronic.

Treatment: — Hot bath, give 1 tablet of Ipecac every half hour, and if vomiting occurs give 1 Opium tablet with the Ipecac until the vomiting stops, then stop the Opium. Give no water for thirst, but give pounded ice. Apply a turpentine poultice over the bowels for a few hours, and follow it with a flaxseed poultice. Send for doctor.

Diarrhoea

Symptoms: — Comes on suddenly, as a rule. Restlessness, disturbed sleep, pain in bowels, vomiting; passages in children, green;

in adults, the color varies. Pain at anus, sour smell, considerable thirst, appetite varies, tongue moist, no tenderness of bowels but considerable wind, no constant fever; may have fast pulse, may have spasm. Moderately dangerous disease.

Treatment: — For children, diet the child, (see Diet), boil the milk and water, if spoon-fed. Give one tablet of Calomel dry to child 1 to 3 years old every hour till 6 are taken, then put 5 tablets of Carbonate of Bismuth in 5 teaspoonfuls of water, with 1 tablet of Opium added, give 1 teaspoonful of this mixture after each passage until the passages are checked. Where there is no pain, leave out the Opium and give one tablet of Carbonate of Bismuth, on the tongue, every hour till passages are checked. For adults, give 1 tablet of Calomel, dry, every half hour until 10 have been taken, then 1 tablet of Opium every 2 hours and 1 tablet of Carbonate of Bismuth every half hour till passages are checked, follow next day with 1 Quinine pill every 3 hours.

Thrush-Sprue

Symptoms: — Comes on in the mouth, may extend down the throat, never attacks the nose or lungs, child becomes fretful, mouth and throat red, inflamed and tender, vomiting and diarrhoea. The Thrush consists of white points at first, which soon run together and become patches, they are slightly elevated, and look like white mould, or curdled milk, after the disease has run on for a short time the patches have a yellowish color, it comes on in young children and is very dangerous unless properly treated. If the previous health of the child is good the case should be cured in 3 to 6 days.

Treatment: — Give good food, (see Diet); dissolve 1 tablet of Sulphate of Zinc in 8 teaspoonfuls of water, and apply this to the throat and mouth with a camel's hair brush or with your finger, do this once a day; twice a day use a little borax in water in the same way; give the child plenty of fresh air, and keep clean by frequent bathing.

Fever and Ague

Symptoms: — Three stages. First stage, cold; the person has a chill which is more or less hard, and lasts a variable length of time; the fingers and lips are blue, teeth chatter, goose pimples appear, pain in back, limbs and head, appetite gone, vomiting or sick stomach common, thirsty, fast breathing, pulse frequent, weak and irregular, may have collapse. Very young children do not have a complete chill. The next stage now sets in. This is called the hot stage, and may come on suddenly or gradually. Skin feels burning hot and dry, is red, may have little rash, face flushed, eyes red, intense thirst, heart and pulse throb, breathing more quiet, headache constant, may be delirious or have spasms This stage lasts from 3 to 8 hours, when the third stage in, which is called the "Sweating Stage." The sweat breaks out first on the forehead and then over the whole body, amount varies, fever falls, breathing becomes easier, the patient falls asleep and awakes in pretty fair health. The Ague may come on every other day, or, every 3 days, and sometimes twice a day. The water is increased during cold and hot stage, but is much lessened in the sweating stage. Ague is not a very fatal disease, but may cause death. It is more fatal to children than grown persons.

Treatment: — During cold stage put the patient in bed, cover up warm, give warm *hot drinks*; if there is much vomiting put 5 tablets of Sulphate of Zinc in 5 teaspoonfuls of water, and give one teaspoonful every 15 minutes till the stomach is well emptied, then stop. This is the dose for a grown person. Give ¼ or ½ teaspoonful to children, according to age. During hot stage give cool drinks and sponge the body with water, to which Vinegar or Alcohol may be added. During sweating stage no remedies are required. Between the stages, when the patient is feeling well, open up the bowels of a grown person by giving 1 to 2 Cathartic pills at night, and follow it next day by a Quinine pill every hour until there is ringing in the ears; for children, open the bowels with a tablet of Calomel every hour till passage is obtained, then give ½ Quinine pill to child 1 to 5 years old every 3 hours; one Quinine pill every 4 hours to child 5 to 10 years old. This disease is apt to become chronic.

Bilious Fever — Remittent Fever

Symptoms: — Green or yellow vomit, loss of appetite, sick stomach, headache, pains over the body, yellow eyeballs, yellow skin, fever which never falls completely, (see Ague) restlessness, constipation, or slimy, green or brown passages, urine scanty and high colored, no regular chill as in ague, hot stage very marked, with extreme thirst; tenderness on the right side, over the liver; white or yellow fur on the tongue, pulse fast, and may be full or irregular; when vomit turns black it is a very dangerous disease, lasts from 1 to 15 days.

Treatment: — Cool drinks, 1 tablet of Calomel every hour for children 1 to 10 years old, and 1 tablet of Calomel every half hour for grown people, until passage of the bowels. If there is no passage 1 hour after 12 tablets of Calomel have been taken, give a dose of Castor Oil or Salts. As soon as the bowels have moved, give 1 Quinine pill every 4 hours to children, every hour to grown people, till eyes are dilated, and pupils large. For the restlessness, put one tablet of Bromide of Potash in 5 teaspoonfuls of water; give 1 teaspoonful every hour to child 1 to 5 years old; two teaspoonfuls every hour to child 5 to 10, and 5 teaspoonfuls every hour to grown person, till quiet. Do not give the Bromide of Potash till after the bowels have moved.

Typhoid Fever

Symptoms: — Comes on slowly, grumbling headache, chilliness with flashes of heat, loss of appetite, sometimes vomiting and sick stomach; by the fifth or sixth day patient goes to bed, may have slight diarrhoea, the fever rises steadily for the first week, then comes the rise and *fall* of the fever, which is characteristic of this disease. The fever in the evening is higher than in the morning, and if you have a thermometer of the kind used by doctors, you will find that this variation is about 2 degrees in the evening and 1 in the morning — that is, it will be 101 in the morning, 103 at night, 102 the next morning, 104 at night. This goes on for about seven days, then for seven days the fever is stationary in morning and evening; say 103 in morning, 105 in evening; then for 7 days the fever falls as it arose, 1 degree a day. Typhoid fever lasts three weeks and cannot be "broken" before that time. The patient is stupid, and out of his head, and has thick, nasty tongue. About the second week mulberry-colored or pinkish spots appear over the body, and stay as long as the fever lasts. There may not be over twenty or thirty of these spots, but you can find them; the teeth become foul, nose-bleed is common; there is pain, on pressure, over the right groin, and the bowels are full of wind; the lips have water blisters over them, the face is pinched, breathing becomes shallow and fast, the pulse is weak and irregular. This disease is very dangerous, is *catching from the passages* from the bowels, which should be thrown into a *disinfectant* as soon as passed. As the patient is subject to relapses, which are more dangerous than the first attack, you should always employ a doctor in this disease.

Treatment: — Put 12 tablets of Carbonate of Ammonia in 8 teaspoonfuls of whisky and give 1 teaspoonful of this every 1, 2 or 3 hours. *Give no fruit, nor food of any kind, except milk.* The greatest danger in Typhoid Fever is the bloody diarrhoea and breaking of the intestines. The disease is bound to run 3 weeks. Keep fever down by sponging the body with alcohol; for thirst give ice to suck, remember the treatment of Typhoid is one of nursing and diet. Keep the patient quiet and allow *no visitors* in the rooms.

N. B. — Do not forget that the passages of the bowels are catching, and should be passed into a vessel which contains a disinfectant.

Inflammation of the Eyes

Symptoms: — Eyes red, painful, swollen, and light hurts them, pain in forehead, water runs from eyes, restless feeling.

Treatment: — Dissolve 1 tablet of Sulphate of Zinc in 8 teaspoonfuls of water and put 2 drops of this mixture in the eye inflamed, twice a day; wash the eyes frequently with hot water. This treatment will cure nearly every eye inflammation; put the medicine into the eye with a teaspoon or dropper.

Inflammation of The Ear

Symptoms: — Intense pain in the ear, deafness on the diseased side, no outward swelling. If child cries suddenly and puts its hand to side of head you can always be certain it has earache.

Treatment: — Ladle hot water into the ear with a tablespoon every hour, put it in as hot as it can be borne and put in at least 12 tablespoonfuls at a time, put on a hot onion poultice when not using water, or blow tobacco smoke in the ear. If matter forms and appears, take the child to your doctor.

Worms

Kinds: — There are 21 kinds. We shall take up two, only, as they are the ones usually found. The first, or round worm, is reddish or reddish-yellow in color, tapers at both ends, and looks like the common earth or "angle" worm; they are prone to move from one place to another in the intestines, and may be found in the stomach. Each female worm lays about 60 million eggs. The thread, maw, or pin worm is white, and looks like a piece of white sewing thread;

they are found in the large intestine and the rectum, where they create intolerable itching. Tape worms inhabit the small intestines, and will not be treated of more fully, as *no one* should try to doctor themselves for their removal, but should go at once to their physician.

Symptoms: — When a child is afflicted with Round Worms, the face will become flushed and then pale, at irregular intervals; color leaden or bluish, lower eyelids swollen, and blue circle around them; thirst, sick stomach, vomiting, appetite variable, breath foul, tongue red and covered with points, pulse fast and irregular, may have spasms, twitching of muscles, disturbed sleep, nightmare, headache, eyes dilated, cross eye, colic, grinding teeth in sleep, generally diarrhoea. The symptoms of thread worm are not so pronounced; there is less fever, colic and nervous symptoms; the itching of the rectum is the most marked and prominent symptoms; the Thread Worm does not kill the patient, the Round Worm may. Never give worm medicine till the child has passed worms, and you have seen them.

Treatment: — Give 1 Santonine tablet and 1 Calomel tablet dry on the tongue three times a day to child 5 years old; at night give castor oil, do this once a week till the worms are expelled. If the child vomits the Santonine, has trouble in seeing or sees things yellow give only ½ tablet of Santonine; you can expel all the common worms in this manner without any danger if you watch the child's seeing powers.

Teething

The first teeth appear at six months, all in at two and one-half years. Second teeth commence at two and one-half years. When gums are painful have them lanced or rub through with some round substance. During teething keep the bowels open and child clean; always a dangerous period of life for sickly children.

Infant Feeding and Diet

Occasionally a mother is unable to suckle her child, and it becomes necessary to bring the child up on the bottle. This is always a dangerous period for children, as the very best of cow's milk is poor for this purpose compared with the mother's milk. Cows which supply milk for infants should be kept clean, and have plenty of air, food and water, and should never be fed on distillery or sugar-house products, neither should they be angered, or heated up by fast driving, but should be kept in the very best possible manner.

Milk used for children should not be acid, and a small amount of lime-water, should be added to it. To make the lime-water, take a piece of un slacked lime as big as an egg, put it in a quart of water, let it settle, then rack off the clear water, and throw away the thick sediment. Put this clear water into a bottle, and when you use it, put 1 tablespoonful into 1 quart of milk. During hot weather, the milk should be boiled and strained before it is fed to the child. For a child under the age of three months, for every three teaspoonfuls of milk, add 1 teaspoonful of water; after 4 months of age, give pure milk; warm it to 98 or 100 degrees before giving; a little sugar of milk can be added to the milk; dissolve it in water before adding. 60 grains of the sugar of milk is enough for ½ pint of milk. Up to 4 months nothing but milk should be given, after that date a little starchy food may be added. This is best given in the form of food for infants found at any drug store. Keep the nursing bottle clean, and on no account give sugar teats or sweet mixtures to infants. Between the ages of 1 and 2 years, a little meat and potato, with bread may be given with milk. Do not "stuff or starve" your child.

Dieting children or grown people consists of cutting of such food or foods as are hurtful. Do not feed in excess, ever; give plain foods, and by plain we mean meats, potatoes, bread, milk and a limited amount of fresh ripe fruit. Pickles, canned fruits, jellies, pies, spices and cakes come under the head of rich foods, and although these will do no harm if taken when the child is well, yet are most emphatically bad when given to the sick. "Water should be given in just large enough quantities to quench thirst. Never allow a sick or convalescent person to eat to excess of even the plainest food; it is better to leave the table hungry than to leave it sleepy and dull. Abstinence in food is as useful and wholesome as abstinence from liquor.

Baths

In giving a hot bath, commence with the water at 90 degrees for adults, and 80 to 85 for children; add hot water until the temperature is 105 for adults, 95 to 100 for children. Wrap a cold cloth around the head and keep it cool while in the bath. A bath, to do any good, should be kept up for at least 1 hour. Mustard or Salt Baths are made by adding Mustard, Common or Sea Salt to the water. Keep clean!

Constipation

Symptoms: — Inability to have *daily* passage of the bowels, when such inability is due to hardness of the matter discharged.
Treatment: — Give injections. (See article on Injections).
All other conditions are treated, in the different diseases.

Injection

It is quite a scientific undertaking to give a good injection. For a common injection for an adult use 1 quart of tepid water, this should be introduced slowly, not in jerks, and after it is all put in, the syringe should be removed and the thumb, covered with a piece of cloth should hold the water in until the inclination to expel it is marked. In introducing the syringe, oil the nozzle well, then put it in very gently, pushing it first a little downward then upward toward the bowels; in an adult it should go in for from 1 ½ to 2 inches, in children from ½ to 1 inch; in children from ½ to 1 pint of water should be used according to age; the water should be made into soap suds with good castile soap.

Boils and Felons

Symptoms: — Local pain, of a sharp, throbbing and knife-like quality; swelling of the part, redness; the redness is localized, or in one spot, matter forms at a longer or shorter interval.

Treatment for Boils: — Paint them with strong Tincture of Iodine, (not in our case, from danger of leakage), give 1 tablet of Muriate of Ammonia on the tongue every hour to grown person, till 12 have been taken; every 2 hours for child 1 to 10 years old, until 6 have been taken; apply hot Flaxseed poultices, and as soon as the Boil is ripe, open it and promote the escape of the matter by poultices; keep the bowels open with Castor Oil or Salts. Do not eat spiced foods or drink any kind of liquor.

Treatment for Felons: — Use the Iodine as in Boils, and put ½ lemon, like a glove-finger, over the Felon. Have it lanced as soon as possible, and have this done even before the matter has completely formed. The lance should be put down to the bone. To prevent irritation from clothing, when boils are not covered by poultices, grease the boil well with Vaseline, and cover with cotton batting, held in place by strips of sticking plaster.

Poultices and Plasters

Mustard Plasters

To make a mustard plaster take 2 tablespoonfuls of best ground mustard, put it into a teacup, add 1 teaspoonful of vinegar, rub this well in, then add hot water by the teaspoonful until paste is formed, take a piece of cloth two inches wider than you want the plaster, and twice as long, spread the mustard on evenly over one-half of this, leaving a margin of 1 inch at end and 1 inch on each side, now fold the clean half like a book cover over the mustard which is spread over the other half, pin or sew the ends and sides and the plaster is finished. When you wish to only have a mild action of the mustard, or for young children, for each teaspoonful of mustard put in 1 teaspoonful of corn meal and leave out the vinegar; do not use flour in place of corn meal, as it cakes. If a mustard plaster is left on too long it will blister.

Turpentine Plaster

To make a Turpentine Stupe or Plaster, fold a piece of flannel in several folds, wring it out of hot water, sprinkle on 10 or 15 drops of Turpentine, apply to the affected spot, and cover with a napkin or towel. Turpentine will blister if left on too long.

Flax-Seed Poultices

To make a Flax-seed Meal Poultice, take 4 or more tablespoon-fuls of Flax-seed Meal, add water to this, rubbing or stirring all the time till you have a rather thin paste; put this in a pan and bring to a boil; have cloth prepared as in mustard plaster; put in the meal, making each poultice 1 inch thick for adults; about as thick as a book cover for young infants, and between these thicknesses for children; make up three, take a colander, put it over a kettle of hot water, put the poultices in the colander, cover them up, and as fast as one cools, draw out the bottom poultice, putting the cool one on top of the second one, which will be the next one you will use; in this manner, by always drawing out the bottom one, you will have a hot, moist poultice without any trouble. As soon as the poultice smells sour, make a new one. Never use poultices after the skin looks white and wrinkled, but apply hot, dry cloths and give the skin a chance to recover its tone.

Charcoal or Yeast Poultices

Are made as above, with the exception that Charcoal or Brewer's Yeast are added to the Flax-seed. Charcoal is used where there is a foul-smelling wound or sore, the Charcoal should be pounded or ground up fine.

Accidents

Bleeding Wounds

Where the accident results in a bleeding wound, if on the legs, feet, arms or hands, and the blood is *bright* red, tie a tight bandage between the body and wound. If the blood is *dark* colored, tie the bandage below the wound, or on the side farthest away from the body. To draw the bandage tight, put a stick through it and twist it up. If the wound is on the body, head or face, fold up five or six pieces of cloth in squares a little larger than the cut or wound, put these pieces of cloth on, one above another, and tie a tight bandage around and over the whole. Before applying these compresses as above, put into the wound 1 to 3 tablets of Tincture of Iron, according to the size of the wound. If the blood comes out in spurts, an artery is cut, and the patient will bleed to death very quickly if you delay in putting on the bandages. When bones are broken, strip off the clothing and put the limbs in as near a natural position as possible. Only a physician should treat broken bones, and you had better send for one at once.

For Burns

Apply moist clay, or paint the parts with Varnish, or dissolve 1 teaspoonful of Baking Powder in a little water and paint the burn with this. In every case of large burns, put cotton wadding over the whole surface to keep out the air. For the pain give an adult 1 Morphine tablet every half hour, till quiet, then stop. For children, dissolve 1 tablet of Morphine in 4 teaspoonfuls of water; give ½ teaspoonful every hour to child 1 to 5 years old; 1 teaspoonful every hour to child 5 to 10 years old till quiet, then stop!

Sunstroke

Is treated by cold applications to head and body, complete rest. The collapse is overcome by giving 1 tablet of Carbonate of Ammonia in 1 teaspoonful of whisky every 10 minutes.

Drowning

Place the drowned person on his back, roll up a coat and put it under the small of the back, then get astride the person facing him now bend down and put your hands around the body one on each side about one inch below the nipple, with the thumbs on or near the breast bone; now raise up and bring the drowned persons body up with you till you have raised him about 3 or 4 inches from the ground, now let him fall back, you making pressure with your thumbs and flat of hand on the chest, still keeping your hands at the back and sides of the body. As soon as you have with your thumbs and flat of hand expelled all the air, count three slowly and go through the same motion again. After 18 or 20 times of this, roll the patient on his side for a moment to allow the water to run from his mouth, then put him on his back again and go through the same performance, do this for at least two hours before you stop, as life has been saved after even longer periods than this. If the drowned person begins to gasp and breathe be careful not to shut off his breath, but help him instead. When breathing is regular put the revived person in bed, wrap up with blankets, put hot jugs or bricks around him and allow him to go to sleep.

Never get excited under any circumstances when there is an accident!

Bruises

Are best treated with cold water, applied often. When a sprain occurs put the joint in *hot* water, and keep it there for at least one hour, adding hot water as required.

Poisons and Their Antidotes

Poisons may be divided into three general classes: Those taken into the stomach by the mouth; those taken into the blood through the skin; and those taken into the lungs through the nose and mouth.

Poisons taken by the mouth are divided into groups or kinds, but all I shall do is to name them and tell you how to save the person poisoned.

Aconite

Symptoms: — Heart beats slower, sweating, urine increased, eyesight dim, pupils of eyes dilated, tongue and breath cold, numbness of hands and feet.

Antidotes: — Heat, brandy, ammonia; put 5 Carbonate of Ammonia tablets in tablespoonful of brandy and give every 15 minutes.

Deadly Night Shade — Belladonna

Symptoms: — Dryness of the throat, blue appearance of lips, diarrhoea, weak heart, red rash like scarlet fever, dilated pupils, headache, delirium, stupor.

Antidote: — Vomit the patient and give Opium; this is all you can do.

Opium — Morphine

Symptoms: — Stupor, snoring, loud breathing, contracted pupils, insensibility to pain, cold hands and feet, blue lips.

Antidote: — Brandy, give hot coffee without milk, electricity, walking, whipping the patient with wet cloths as he is led around, give Belladonna, vomit the patient with Sulphate of Zinc.

Arsenic

Symptoms:— Pain in bowels, vomiting, bloody mucus, increase flow of spittle, sickness of the stomach, bloody diarrhoea, irritable heart, swelling of eyelids with general swelling of body, limbs, hands and feet; trembling, dryness of the mouth, great thirst, bowels drawn in, collapse.

Antidote: — Give Sesquioxide of Iron, 8 grains to each grain of Arsenic swallowed. Send for your doctor.

Strychnine

Symptoms: — Shocks or twitching runs through the muscles, limbs drawn up, head thrown back during spasms, which comes on suddenly; the buzzing of a fly, or breath of cold air, will throw patient into spasms face grins and badly drawn up, foam flies from lips, body curves in a bow backward, skin blue, passage of water and of bowels, during intervals between spasms, patient is conscious, mind is clear until death.

Antidote: — Vomit the patient and put asleep with chloroform. Usually die, no matter what is done.

Mercury — Corrosive Sublimate

Symptoms: — Vomiting of bloody mucus, pain in stomach and bowels, cramps, purging, collapse, with weak heart and blue skin.

Antidote: — Wheat flour, white of egg, lime-water milk and vomit the patient.

Oxalic Acid

Symptoms: — Death in 10 minutes has resulted from a large dose of this poison. Horrible pain in stomach and bowels, bloody vomit. Oxalic Acid looks like Epsom Salts.

Antidote: — Vomit the patient, give lime-water, white, of egg, flaxseed tea, flour and starch.

The second group of poisons are snake and animal bites, bee and insect stings.

Treatment: — Burn out the wound at once with burning match or hot iron, tie a tight bandage between the wound and body, if on the limbs

For snake bites dissolve 12 Carbonate of Ammonia tablets in 1 pint of whisky or brandy and drink it all, repeat this till patient is drunk.

For bee or other stings, apply moist wet clay to the sting.

The third group will include Chloroform, Aether and Coal Gas.

Treatment: — For Chloroform stand the patient on his or her head, give Carbonate of Ammonia 12 tablets in ½ pint of whisky and whip the patient with cold wet cloths, give artificial respiration or breathing.

For Aether give the whisky and Carbonate of Ammonia, artificial breathing and whipping.

For Coal Gas, fresh air, artificial breathing and whisky as soon as the patient can swallow.

Hints for The Sick Room

Never whisper or talk loud, wear slippers, and clothes that do not crackle. Keep the room clean and well ventilated; to ventilate a room, open the top of the window, now take a board about 8 inches wide, that will just fit between the sides of the window at the bottom, raise the lower sash 6 inches, put this board up, leaving 1 inch space between it and the window proper; in this way air can enter the room without creating a draught. Never bring a large quantity of food to a sick person; it is better to make three trips to the kitchen than to sicken your patient; put the food on a tray and serve as daintily as you can, treat your sick as if they were honored guests, and get out your prettiest dishes. Make the sick-room. as cheerful as you can, remove all birds and animals; keep the house quiet; have all flights shaded; do not leave medicines where the patient can get at them; you cannot always tell what might happen if you let a sick person "dose" himself.

Humor the delusions of the sick, be firm but never scold or find fault or tell how tired you are, don't talk about the patient in his or her hearing, never go outside the door with the doctor; prepare the medicines where the patient can see you, but not what you are doing, in other words, turn your back; *allow no visitors* in the room, change the pillows often, keep the bed clean, wash the face and hands of the sick often, don't allow your own to smell of the cooking or anything else. Don't fuss around the room; when you have anything to do, do it, and then sit down; don't take your sewing into the room, as it will drive some people into a fever, be kind, be careful and do just as the doctor tells you to, don't know too much.

Our Household Medicine Case

(Advertisement)

Contains the following Medicines:

	Each Tablet Contains:
1 Aconite,	1 drop
2 Bromide of Potash,	5 grains
3 Belladonna,	1½ drop
4 Ipecac,	¼ grain
5 Calomel,	1-10 grain
6 Carbonate of Bismuth,	1 grain
7 Carbonate of Ammonia,	1 grain
8 Cathartic Pills,	Vegetable
9 Chlorate of Potash,	1 grain
10 Digitalis,	2 drops
11 Morphine,	1-12 grain
12 Muriate of Ammonia,	1 grain
13 Opium,	¼ grain
14 Quinine Pills,	1 grain
15 Sulphur,	2 grains
16 Santonine,	¼ grain
17 Sulphate of Zinc,	1 grain
18 Tincture of Iron,	5 drops

Don't get out of Medicine!

Any bottle in this case refilled by us for 15 cts, and medicines sent postpaid, without delay, on receipt of order accompanied by the cash.

Full directions for treating any of the common diseases with the above Medicines, will be found in "Our Family Doctor," which accompanies this case. The Medicines are measured and compounded with scientific accuracy, and are of the very first quality, and strictly pure, as the following affidavit shows:

Offices of Frederick Stearns & Co.,
Detroit, Mich., U. S. A.

Frederick K. Stearns, President of the corporation of Frederick Stearns & Co., being duly sworn, deposes and says that the said corporation do a manufacturing business in the city of Detroit, and State of Michigan, and that they put up and furnish by contract the medicines used by the Detroit Medicine Company of said city and State, and sold by the said last named company, by subscription, in a package known as **"Our Household Medicine Case,"** and that the said medicines are made from strictly pure drugs, and are of the best quality in every respect.

(Signed) **Frederick K. Stearns.**

Taken, subscribed and sworn to before me, a Notary Public, in and for the County of Wayne and State of Michigan, this 12th day of July, A D. 1887.

M. L. Dunning,
Notary Public, Wayne Co., Mich.

www.ingramcontent.com/pod-product-compliance
Lightning Source LLC
Chambersburg PA
CBHW022056190326
41520CB00008B/790